Keto Crockpot Cookbook For Beginners

Cook While Learning! 50+ Quick And Easy Healthy Keto Recipes For Absolute Beginners. Get Creative And Start Your Diet Today!

Lillie L. Carter

Table of Contents:

KETO CROCKPOT COOKBOOK FOR BEGINNERS

Zucchini Lasagna with Minced Pork

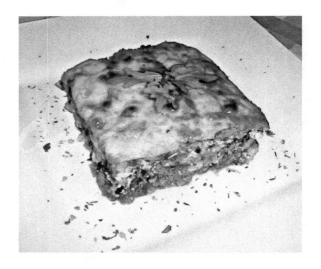

Preparation Time: 20 minutes

Cooking Time: 8 hours

Servings: 6

Ingredients:

4 medium-sized zucchini

1 small onion, diced

1 garlic clove, minced

2 cups lean ground pork, minced

2 regular cans diced Italian tomatoes

2 Tablespoons olive oil

2 cups grated Mozzarella cheese

1 egg

Small bunch of fresh basil or 1 Tablespoon dry basil

Salt and pepper to taste

2 Tablespoons butter to grease crock-pot

Directions:

Cut the zucchini lengthwise making 6 slices from each vegetable. Salt and let drain. Discard the liquid.

In a pan, heat the olive oil. Sauté the onion and garlic for 5 minutes.

Add minced meat and cook for another 5 minutes. Add tomatoes and simmer for another 5 minutes.

Add seasoning and mix well. Add basil leaves. Cool slightly.

Beat the egg, mix in 1 cup of cheese.

Grease the crock-pot with butter and start layering the lasagna. First, the zucchini slices, then a layer of meat mixture, top it with cheese, and repeat. Finish with zucchini and the second cup of cheese.

Cover, cook on low for 8 hours.

Nutrition:

Carbs: 10g

Protein: 23g

Fiber: 39g

Chili Con Steak

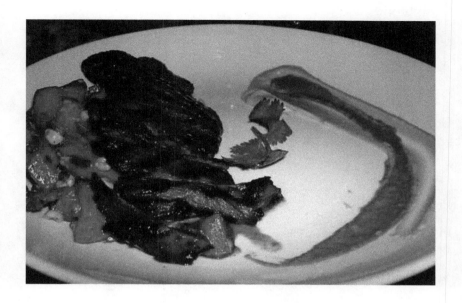

Preparation Time: 5 minutes

Cooking Time: 6 hours on high

Servings: 6

Ingredients:

3 pounds beef steak, cubed

1 Tablespoon paprika

½ teaspoon chili powder

1 teaspoon dried oregano

½ teaspoon ground cumin

Salt and pepper to taste

4 Tablespoons butter

½ cup sliced leeks

2 cups Italian diced tomatoes

1 cup broth, beef

Directions:

Place all the ingredients in the crock-pot by order on list.

Stir together.

Cover, cook on high for 6 hours.

Nutrition:

Carbs: 9g

Protein: 62g

Fiber: 26g

One-Pot Chicken and Green Beans

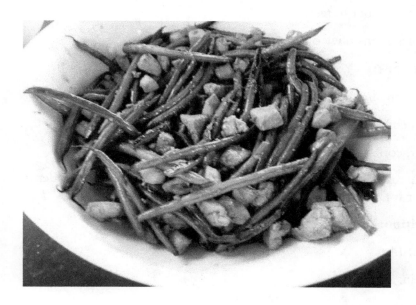

Preparation Time: 5 minutes

Cooking Time: 8 hours

Servings: 6

Ingredients:

2 cups green beans, trimmed

2 large beef tomatoes, diced

1 red onion, diced

2 garlic cloves, minced

1 bunch chopped fresh dill (around ⅛ cup)

1 lemon, juiced

4 Tablespoons butter

1 cup chicken broth

6 chicken thighs, skin on

Salt and pepper to taste

2 Tablespoons olive oil

Directions:

Add all the ingredients to the crock-pot in order on list.

Brush chicken thighs with olive oil; season with salt and pepper.

Cover, cook on low for 8 hours.

When ready, if desired, take the chicken out and crisp it under a broiler for few minutes.

Nutrition:

Carbs: 14g

Protein: 26g

Fiber: 24g

Two-Meat Chili

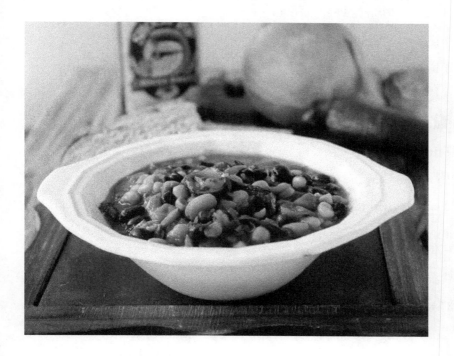

Preparation Time: 15 minutes

Cooking Time: 6 hours and 30 minutes

Servings: 6

Ingredients:

1 ½ cups lean ground pork sausage meat

1 ¾ cups stewing beef, cubed

2 Tablespoons olive oil

1 bell pepper, sliced

1 white onion, sliced in semi-circles

1 cup beef broth

2 Tablespoons tomato paste

2 Tablespoons sweet paprika

1 teaspoon chili powder

1 teaspoon cumin

1 teaspoon oregano

Salt and pepper to taste

Directions:

In a pan, heat the olive oil. Brown the beef, transfer to the crock-pot.

Then, brown the sausage and transfer to crock-pot.

In the same pan, sweat the onion and pepper slices for 4-5 minutes, pour over the meat.

Add remaining ingredients to crock-pot.

Cover, cook on low for 6 hours.

Turn to high, remove the lid and let the liquid reduce for 30 minutes.

Nutrition:

Carbs: 10g

Protein: 28g

Fiber: 48g

Pork Curry

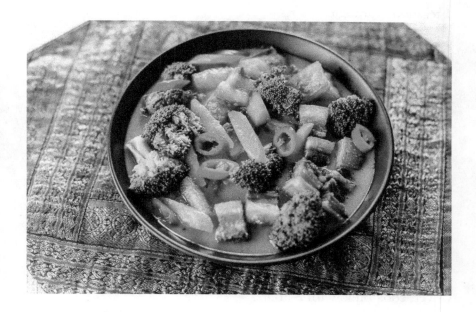

Preparation Time: 10 minutes

Cooking Time: 8 hours

Servings: 6

Ingredients:

2.2 pounds pork shoulder, cubed

1 Tablespoon coconut oil

1 yellow onion, diced

2 garlic cloves, minced

2 Tablespoons tomato paste

1 small can coconut milk – 12 fl ounces

1 cup water

½ cup white wine

1 teaspoon turmeric

1 teaspoon ginger powder

1 teaspoon curry powder

½ teaspoon paprika

Salt and pepper to taste

Directions:

In a pan, heat 1 tablespoon olive oil. Sauté the onion and garlic for 2-3 minutes.

Add the pork and brown it. Finish with tomato paste.

In the crock-pot, mix all remaining ingredients, submerge the meat in the liquid.

Cover, cook on low for 8 hours.

Nutrition:

Carbs: 7g

Protein: 30g

Fiber: 34g

Homemade Vegetable Stock

Preparation Time: 30 minutes

Cooking Time: 12 hours

Servings: 4

Ingredients:

4 quarts cold filtered water

12 whole peppercorns

3 peeled and chopped carrots

3 chopped celery stalks

2 bay leaves

4 smashed garlic cloves

1 large quartered onion

2 tablespoons apple cider vinegar

Any other vegetable scraps

Directions:

Put everything in your slow cooker and cover.

Do not turn on; let it sit for 30 minutes.

When that's done, cook on low for 12 hours.

Strain the broth and discard the solids.

Before using, keep the stock in a container in the fridge for 2-3 hours.

Stock will keep fresh for 4-5 days, or frozen indefinitely.

Nutritional Info (1 cup per serving):

Total calories: 11

Protein: 0

Carbs: 3

Fat: 0

Fiber: 0

Cream of Zucchini Soup

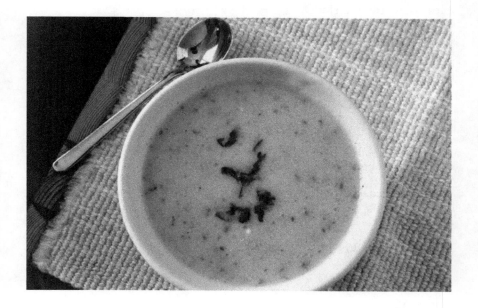

Preparation Time: 10 minutes

Cooking Time: 2 hours

Servings: 4

Ingredients:

3 cups vegetable stock

2 pounds chopped zucchini

2 minced garlic cloves

¾ cup chopped onion

¼ cup basil leaves

1 tablespoon extra-virgin olive oil

Salt and pepper to taste

Directions:

Heat olive oil in a skillet.

When hot, cook garlic and onion for about 5 minutes.

Pour into your slow cooker with the rest of the ingredients.

Close the lid.

Cook on low for 2 hours.

When time is up, puree the soup with an immersion blender, or in batches in a regular blender.

Taste and season more if needed!

Nutrition:

Total calories: 96

Protein: 7

Carbs: 11

Fat: 5

Fiber: 2.3

Vegetable Korma (Stew)

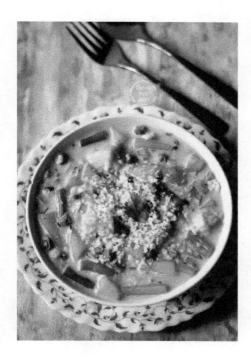

Preparation Time: 5 minutes

Cooking Time: 8 hours

Servings: 4

Ingredients:

1 head's worth of cauliflower florets

¾ of a 10-ounce can of full-fat coconut milk

2 cups chopped green beans

½ chopped onion

2 minced garlic cloves

2 tablespoons curry powder

2 tablespoons coconut flour

1 teaspoon garam masala

Salt and pepper to taste

Directions:

Add vegetables into your slow cooker.

Mix coconut milk with seasonings.

Pour into the slow cooker.

Sprinkle over coconut flour and mix until blended.

Close the lid.

Cook on low for 8 hours.

Taste and season more if necessary.

Serve!

Nutrition:

Total calories: 206

Protein: 5

Carbs: 18

Fat: 14

Fiber: 9.5

Zoodles w/ Cauliflower-Tomato Sauce

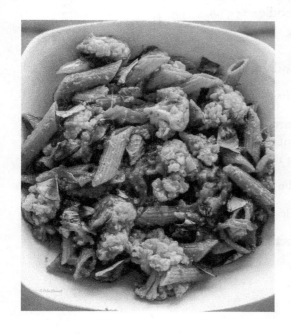

Preparation Time: 30 minutes

Cooking Time: 3 hours

Servings: 4

Ingredients:

5 large spiralized zucchinis (or julienned zucchinis)

Two 24-ounce cans of diced tomatoes

2 small heads' worth of cauliflower florets

1 cup diced sweet onion

4 minced garlic cloves

½ cup veggie broth

5 teaspoons Italian seasoning

18

Salt and pepper to taste

Enough water to cover zoodles

Directions:

Put everything but the zoodles into your slow cooker.

Cook on high for 3 ½ hours.

When time is up, smash into a chunky sauce with a potato masher or another utensil. If you want a smooth sauce, puree with an immersion blender, or in batches in a regular blender.

To cook the zoodles, boil a large pot of water.

When boiling, cook zoodles for just 1 minute, then drain.

Season with salt and pepper.

Serve sauce over zoodles!

Nutrition:

Total calories: 113

Protein: 7

Carbs: 22

Fat: 2

Fiber: 10.5

Spaghetti Squash Carbonara

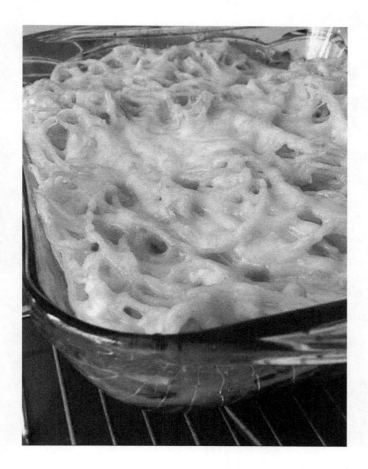

Preparation Time: 10 minutes

Cooking Time: 8 hours

Servings: 4

Ingredients:

2 cups water

One 3-pound spaghetti squash

½ cup coconut bacon

½ cup fresh spinach leaves

1 egg

3 tablespoons heavy cream

3 tablespoons unsweetened almond milk

½ cup grated Parmesan cheese

1 teaspoon garlic powder

Salt and pepper to taste

Directions:

Put squash in your cooker and pour in 2 cups of water.

Close the lid.

Cook on low for 8-9 hours.

When the spaghetti squash cools, mix egg, cream, milk, and cheese in a bowl.

When the squash is cool enough for you to handle with oven mitts, cut it open lengthwise and scrape out noodles.

Mix in the egg mixture right away.

Add spinach and seasonings.

Top with coconut bacon and enjoy!

Nutrition:

Total calories: 211

Protein: 5

Carbs: 26

Fat: 11

Fiber: 5.1

Summery Bell Pepper + Eggplant Salad

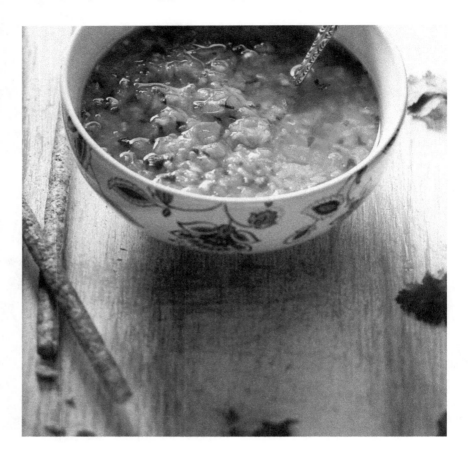

Preparation Time: 15 minutes

Cooking Time: 8 hours

Servings: 4

Ingredients:

One 24-ounce can of whole tomatoes

2 sliced yellow bell peppers

2 small eggplants (smaller ones tend to be less bitter)

1 sliced red onion

1 tablespoon paprika

2 teaspoons cumin

Salt and pepper to taste

Squeeze of lime juice

Directions:

Mix all the ingredients in your slow cooker.

Close the lid.

Cook on low for 7-8 hours.

When time is up, serve warm, or chill in the fridge for a few hours before eating.

Nutrition:

Total calories: 128

Protein: 5

Carbs: 27

Fat: 1

Fiber: 9.7

Cheesy Creamy Cauliflower Mash

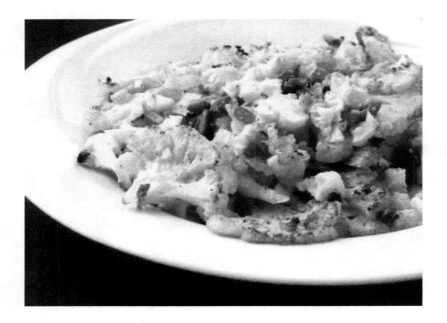

Preparation Time: 10 minutes

Cooking Time: 3 hours

Servings: 6

Ingredients:

1 large head's worth of cauliflower florets

4-ounces full-fat sour cream

1 cup shredded cheddar cheese

3 tablespoons grass-fed butter

2 tablespoons chopped scallions

¼ teaspoon garlic powder

Salt and pepper to taste

Handful of coconut bacon

Enough water to cover cauliflower

Directions:

Put cauliflower florets in your slow cooker.

Pour in enough water to cover.

Close the lid.

Cook on high for 3 hours.

When time is up, puree with an immersion blender or in batches with a regular blender.

Fold in sour cream, butter, and cheese to melt.

When combined, add seasonings.

Serve with coconut bacon on top!

Nutrition:

Total calories: 159

Protein: 5

Carbs: 7

Fat: 13

Fiber: 3.5

Creamy Chicken Soup

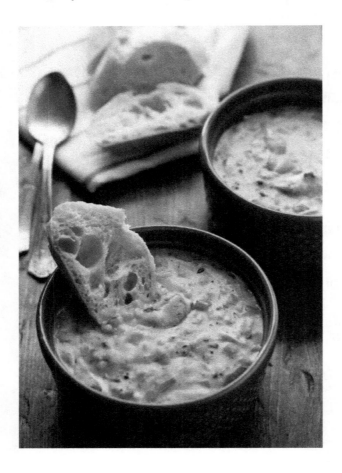

Preparation Time: 10 minutes

Cooking Time: 8 hours

Servings: 4

Ingredients:

3 cooked + shredded chicken breasts

4 cups chicken stock

1 cup heavy cream

2 chopped carrots

2 chopped celery stalks

1 diced sweet onion

2 minced garlic cloves

1 teaspoon dried thyme

Salt and pepper to taste

Directions:

Put all the ingredients (except cream) into your slow cooker.

Cook on low for 8 hours.

When there are thirty minutes left to go, add cream.

When time is up, taste and season more with salt and pepper if needed.

Serve hot!

Nutrition:

Total calories: 123

Protein: 16

Carbs: 10

Fat: 3

Fiber: 1

Mexican Chicken Soup

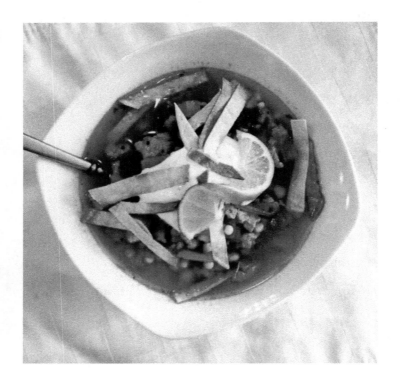

Preparation Time: 10 minutes

Cooking Time: 2 hours

Servings: 4

Ingredients:

32-ounces chicken broth

One 28-ounce can of tomatoes

2 chopped cooked chicken breasts

2 seeded and diced jalapeno peppers

1 cup water

1 chopped red onion

4 minced garlic cloves

2 tablespoons no-sugar tomato paste

1 handful of chopped parsley

1 teaspoon cumin

½ teaspoon chili powder

Drizzle of olive oil

Salt and pepper to taste

Directions:

Pour oil into a skillet and heat.

When hot, add ¼ cup broth, jalapenos, onion, garlic, salt, and pepper.

When the onions and peppers are soft, pour into the slow cooker.

Pour in the rest of the ingredients, except parsley.

Close the lid.

Cook on low for 2 hours.

Chicken should be 165-degrees and very tender.

Shred chicken and serve!

Nutrition:

Total calories: 135

Protein: 13

Carbs: 20

Fat: 3

Fiber: 2.5

Thai-Inspired Chicken Soup

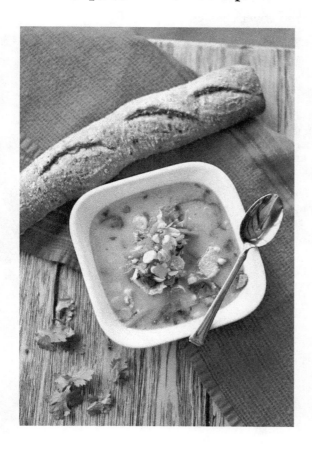

Preparation Time: 10 minutes

Cooking Time: 8 hours

Servings: 8

Ingredients:

1 whole organic chicken

One 14-ounce can of full-fat coconut milk

4-inch thumb of chopped ginger

1 chopped lemongrass stalk

Enough vegetable broth to cover chicken

Splash of Red Boat fish sauce

Salt to taste

Directions:

Put the whole chicken, ginger, and lemongrass in your slow cooker.

Pour in coconut milk, and enough vegetable broth to cover chicken.

Close the lid.

Cook on low for 8-10 hours.

When time is up, remove the chicken, and pull all the meat off the bones.

Return meat to the soup.

Taste, and season with salt and fish sauce as needed.

Serve!

Nutrition:

Total calories: 330

Protein: 22

Carbs: 2

Fat: 26

Fiber: 0

Spicy Pepper Chicken Soup

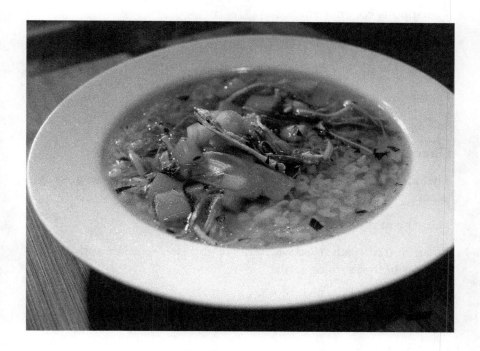

Preparation Time: 20 minutes

Cooking Time: 8 hours

Servings: 6

Ingredients:

3 chopped raw chicken breasts

8-ounces chicken stock

2 seeded and chopped jalapeno peppers

1 chopped poblano chili pepper

½ cup chopped green onions

3 minced garlic cloves

5 teaspoons 100% natural peanut butter

4 teaspoons coconut aminos

4 teaspoons lime juice

½ tablespoon+ crushed red pepper flakes

1 teaspoon ground ginger

Salt and pepper to taste

Directions:

The night before you plan on making the soup, put all the ingredients (minus green onions) in your slow cooker.

Marinate in the fridge overnight.

When you're ready to cook, remove the slow cooker and wait 20 minutes before turning it on.

Turn to low and cook for 6-8 hours.

Taste and add more red pepper flakes if you want more heat.

Garnish with chopped green onions and serve!

Nutrition:

Total calories: 102

Protein: 13

Carbs: 4

Fat: 4

Fiber: 0

Turkey + Herbs Soup

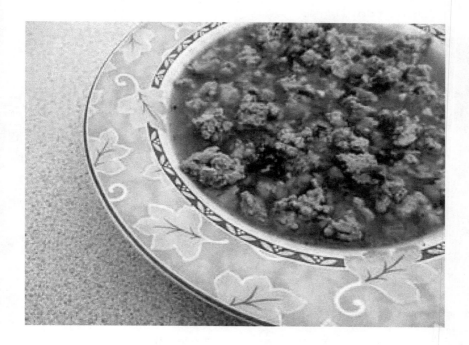

Preparation Time: 10 minutes

Cooking Time: 2 hours

Servings: 4

Ingredients:

4 cups turkey/chicken stock

3 cups cooked turkey meat

3 cups chopped fresh spinach

1 cup chopped onion

2 fresh rosemary sprigs

½ tablespoon grass-fed butter

1 teaspoon garlic powder

½ teaspoon dried parsley

½ teaspoon dried thyme

Salt and pepper to taste

Directions:

Melt the butter in a skillet and add onions.

Cook until soft.

Add to your slow cooker with the rest of the ingredients (except spinach).

Close the lid.

Cook for 2 hours on low. Since there isn't anything raw in the recipe, you're basically just simmering the flavors together.

A few minutes before serving, stir in the spinach, and let the heat of the soup wilt the greens.

Taste and season with more salt and pepper if needed.

Enjoy!

Nutrition:

Total calories: 331

Protein: 19

Carbs: 6

Fat: 26

Fiber: 0

Beefy Chili

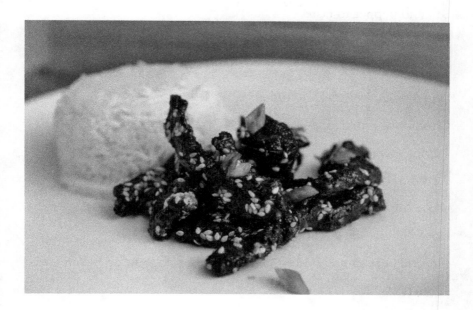

Preparation Time: 10 minutes

Cooking Time: 6 hours

Servings: 6

Ingredients:

21-ounces ground beef

21-ounces stew beef

One 8-ounce can of diced tomatoes

1 cup beef stock

2 chopped sweet onions

4 minced garlic cloves

1 tablespoon red chili flakes

Splash of extra virgin olive oil

Salt and pepper to taste

Directions:

Heat olive oil in a skillet.

When hot, add garlic and onions.

Cook until softened.

Put into your slow cooker.

Add the rest of the ingredients.

Close the lid.

Cook on low for 4-6 hours.

Ground beef should be 160-degrees, while steak can be 145-degrees.

Serve hot!

Nutrition:

Total calories: 325

Protein: 40

Carbs: 6

Fat: 16

Fiber: 0

Crack Chicken

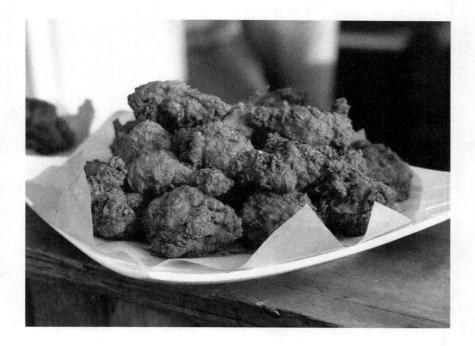

Preparation Time: 15 minutes

Cooking Time: 8 hours

Servings: 2

Ingredients:

1 chicken breast

1 packet of Ranch dressing

4 oz. cream cheese

2 slices bacon, cooked and crumbled

Directions:

Put the chicken breast in the crockpot.

Pour the dressing in and add the cream cheese.

Cover and cook for 8 hours on low.

Mix in the crumbled bacon when cooked.

Nutrition:

Calories: 410

Fat: 32 g

Net carbs: 4 g

Protein: 28 g

Salsa Chicken

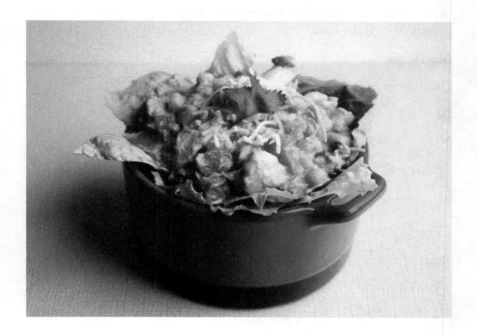

Preparation Time: 15 minutes

Cooking Time: 2 hours

Servings: 2

Ingredients:

1 chicken breast

1/2 cup fresh salsa

1/2 cup shredded cheese

Directions:

Lightly grease your crockpot with olive oil.

Place the chicken breast in the crockpot and pour the salsa over it.

Cover and cook for 2 hours on high.

When cook, top with cheese and bake for 15 minutes in a preheated oven to 425 F degrees.

Nutrition:

Calories: 398

Fat: 18.3 g

Net carbs: 4.2 g

Protein: 42.9 g

Chicken Tikka Masala

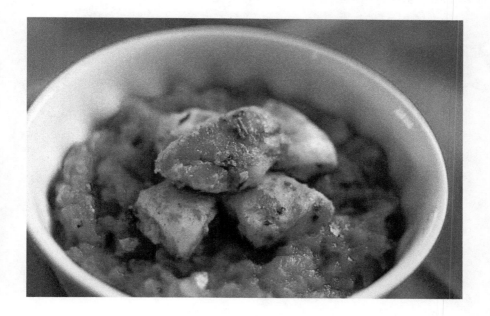

Preparation Time: 15 minutes

Cooking Time: 6 hours

Servings: 2

Ingredients:

1 lb. chicken thighs, de-boned and chopped into bite-size

3 tsp Garam Masala

5 oz. diced tomatoes

1/2 cup heavy cream

1/2 cup coconut milk

Directions:

Put chicken to crockpot and add grated ginger knob on top.

Also add the seasonings: 1 tsp onion powder, 2 minced cloves of garlic, 1 tsp paprika and 2 tsp salt. Mix.

Add tomatoes and coconut oil. Mix.

Cook for 6 hours on low.

When cooked, add heavy cream to thicken the curry.

Nutrition:

Calories: 493

Fat: 41.2 g

Net carbs: 5.8 g

Protein: 46 g

Lemongrass and Coconut Chicken Drumsticks

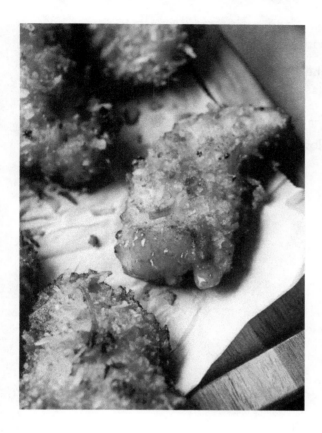

Preparation Time: 15 minutes

Cooking Time: 5 hours

Servings: 2

Ingredients:

5 chicken drumsticks, skinless

1 stalk lemongrass, rough bottom removed

1/2 cup coconut milk

1/2 tbsp coconut aminos

Directions:

Season drumsticks with salt and pepper. Place in the crockpot.

In a blender, mix the lemongrass, coconut milk, coconut aminos, garlic and ginger to taste, 1 tbsp fish sauce and desired spices.

Pour the mixture over the drumsticks.

Cover and cook on low for 5 hours.

Nutrition:

Calories: 460

Fat: 39.7 g

Net carbs: 4.7 g

Protein: 36 g

Bacon & Chicken

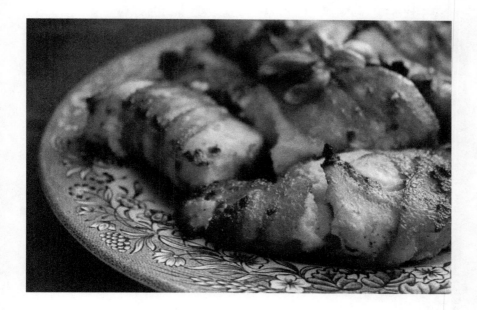

Preparation Time: 5 minutes

Cooking Time: 8 hours

Servings: 2

Ingredients:

1 chicken breasts

4 slices of bacon, sliced

2 tbsp. dried thyme

1 tbsp. dried oregano

1 tbsp. dried rosemary

Directions:

Mix all ingredients in the crockpot. Add salt to taste.

Cook for 8 hours on low.

Nutrition:

Calories: 460

Fat: 39.7 g

Net carbs: 4.7 g

Protein: 36 g

Roasted Chicken with Lemon & Parsley Butter

Preparation Time: 5 minutes

Cooking Time: 8 hours

Servings: 2

Ingredients:

4 lb. chicken, any part

1 whole lemon, sliced

2 tbsp. butter or ghee

1 tbsp. parsley, chopped

Directions:

Rub chicken all over with salt and pepper to taste. Put it in the crockpot and pour 1 cup of water.

Cover and cook for 3 hours on high.

When cooked, add the lemon slices butter and parsley to the crockpot.

Cook and cover for another 10 minutes.

Nutrition:

Calories: 300

Fat: 18 g

Net carbs: 1 g

Protein: 29 g

Onion and Mushroom Chicken Breasts

Preparation Time: 5 minutes

Cooking Time: 8 hours

Servings: 2

Ingredients:

1 sliced onions

1 cup sliced mushrooms

2 chicken breasts

1 cup chicken broth

Thyme

Directions:

Place the half the onion slices on the bottom of the crockpot and add the chicken on top.

Top again with the remainder of onion slices.

Add all other ingredients carefully into the crockpot. Add salt and pepper to taste.

Cook on low for 8 hours.

Nutrition:

Calories: 345

Fat: 29 g

Net carbs: 4 g

Protein: 32 g

Turkey-Stuffed Peppers

Preparation Time: 15 minutes

Cooking Time: 8 hours

Servings: 2

Ingredients:

1/2 lb. turkey, ground

2 whole green bell peppers, top cut off and insides scraped off

12 oz. jar tomato sauce

Directions:

Mix turkey, 1 tbsp. tomato sauce and onion and garlic to taste in a bowl.

Separate mixture into two parts and put them inside the peppers.

Place the stuffed peppers in the crockpot and add the remaining tomato sauce.

Add 1/4 cup of water.

Cover and cook for 8 hours on low.

Nutrition:

Calories: 422

Fat: 27.5 g

Net carbs: 3.6 g

Protein: 30.8 g

Creamy Mexican Chicken

Preparation Time: 5 minutes

Cooking Time: 6 hours

Servings: 2

Ingredients:

1/3 cup sour cream

1/4 cup chicken stock

7 oz diced tomatoes

1/2 pack taco seasoning

1 lb. chicken breast

Directions:

In the crockpot, mix all ingredients until well combined.

Cover and cook for 6 hours on low.

Nutrition:

Calories: 262

Fat: 13 g

Net carbs: 5.8 g

Protein: 32 g

Salsa Chicken with Lime and Mozzarella

Preparation Time: 15 minutes

Cooking Time: 2 hours

Servings: 2

Ingredients:

1 cup simmered salsa

2 chicken breasts, skinned and trimmed lengthwise

1 tbsp. lime juice

1/2 cup low-fat Mozzarella, grated

Directions:

Put chicken in the crockpot. Season with salt, garlic and pepper to taste.

Pour the salsa and lime juice into the crockpot.

Cover and cook for 2 hours on high.

When cooked, transfer the chicken to a casserole dish and top with the salsa in the crockpot.

Sprinkle the Mozzarella.

Put on broiler for 5 minutes.

Nutrition:

Calories: 307

Fat: 21 g

Net carbs: 3.8 g

Protein: 29 g

BBQ Bacon Chicken

Preparation Time: 5 minutes

Cooking Time: 6 hours 30 minutes

Servings: 2

Ingredients:

2 chicken breasts, thawed

10 oz. barbecue sauce

1/4 tbsp. liquid smoke

8 oz. bacon, cooked and chopped

Directions:

Cook chicken in crockpot for 6 hours on low.

When cooked, drain all liquids and add all other ingredients.

Cook for another 30 minutes on high.

Nutrition:

Calories: 401

Fat: 18 g

Net carbs: 5.7 g

Protein: 50 g

Bacon-Wrapped Turkey Breast with Tomatoes

Preparation Time: 10 minutes

Cooking Time: 8 hours

Servings: 2

Ingredients:

1/2 lb. turkey breast

4 oz. bacon, sliced and cooked

2 tomatoes, diced

Bay leaves to taste

Directions:

Combine tomatoes and bay leaves in the crockpot, together with 1/4 tsp each of garlic powder and black pepper.

Wrap the turkey breasts with bacon and add them into the crockpot.

Cover and cook for 8 hours on low.

Nutrition:

Calories: 421

Fat: 29 g

Net carbs: 4.3 g

Protein: 48 g

Peach Chipotle Chicken

Preparation Time: 5 minutes

Cooking Time: 6 hours 30 minutes

Servings: 2

Ingredients:

2 chicken breasts, skinless and thawed

10 oz. Chipotle Barbecue Sauce

10 oz. peach, sliced

Directions:

Cook chicken in crockpot for 6 hours on low.

When cooked, drain all liquids and add all other ingredients.

Cook for another 30 minutes on high.

Nutrition:

Calories: 425

Fat: 29.7 g

Net carbs: 3.6 g

Protein: 36.8 g

Green Chili Chicken

Preparation Time: 10 minutes

Cooking Time: 6 hours 30 minutes

Servings: 2

Ingredients:

2 chicken thighs, thawed

2 oz green chili

1 tsp garlic salt

Directions:

Place chicken in the crockpot and cook for 6 hours on low.

Drain the juices afterwards and add in the other two ingredients.

Cover and cook for another 30 minutes on high.

Shred chicken with a fork.

Nutrition:

Calories: 347

Fat: 23.8 g

Net carbs: 3.7 g

Protein: 33.1 g

Chicken Picatta

Preparation Time: 10 minutes

Cooking Time: 3 hours

Servings: 2

Ingredients:

2 chicken breasts

1/4 cup tomatoes, diced

2 tbsp. melted butter

7 oz. artichoke hearts, quartered

Directions:

Except for the parmesan, combine all ingredients in the crockpot, including garlic cloves and pepper to taste.

Cook on high for 3 hours.

Top with parmesan cheese.

Nutrition:

Calories: 343

Fat: 29 g

Net carbs: 6 g

Protein: 37 g

Beef Taco Meat

Preparation Time: 10 minutes

Cooking Time: 45 minutes

Servings: 10

Ingredients:

2 pounds of ground beef

2 tablespoons of butter

3 teaspoons of ground cumin

2 teaspoons of garlic powder

2 teaspoons of paprika

1 teaspoon of salt

1 teaspoon of onion powder

½ teaspoon of black pepper

1/8 teaspoon of cayenne pepper

Directions:

Press "Sautee/Browning" button on the Crock-Pot Express and add the butter.

Once hot, add the ground beef and cook until brown, breaking up using a durable metal or wooden spoon.

Add the ground cumin, garlic powder, paprika, salt, onion powder, black pepper, and cayenne pepper. Stir until well combined.

Turn off "Sautee/Browning" button on the Crock-Pot Express.

Serve and enjoy!

Nutrition:

Calories: 130

Fat: 4g

Carbohydrates: 1g

Dietary Fiber: 0g

Protein: 19g

Desirable Beef Curry Stew

Preparation Time: 5 minutes

Cooking Time: 45 minutes

Servings: 6

Ingredients:

2 ½ pounds of beef stew chunks

1 pound of broccoli florets

3 zucchinis, chopped

½ cup of chicken broth

2 tablespoons of curry powder

1 tablespoon of garlic powder

2 teaspoons of salt

1 (14-ounce) can of coconut milk

Directions:

Add all the ingredients except for the coconut milk to the Crock-Pot Express and stir until well combined.

Lock the lid and ensure the valve is closed.

Press the "Meat/Stew" button and set the time for 45 minutes.

When the cooking is done, naturally release the pressure and remove the lid.

Stir the coconut milk to the curry and adjust the seasoning as needed.

Serve and enjoy!

Nutrition:

Calories: 490

Fat: 30g

Carbohydrates: 8g

Dietary Fiber: 3g

Protein: 40g

Balsamic Pot Roast

Preparation Time: 10 minutes

Cooking Time: 4 hours

Servings: 10

Ingredients:

1 (3-pound) boneless chuck roast

2 tablespoons of olive oil

1 tablespoon of salt

1 teaspoon of black pepper

1 teaspoon of garlic powder

¼ cup of balsamic vinegar

2 cups of water

½ cup of onions, chopped

¼ teaspoon of xanthan gum

1 tablespoon of fresh parsley, chopped

Directions:

Season the chuck roast with salt, black pepper, and garlic powder.

Press the "Saute/Browning" button on the Crock-Pot Express and add the olive oil.

Once hot, add the chuck roast and cook until brown. Deglaze the Crock-Pot Express with the balsamic vinegar and cook for an additional minute.

Add the water and onions to the Crock-Pot Express and bring to a boil.

Lock the lid and ensure the valve is closed.

64

Press the "Slow Cook" button and set the time to 4 hours.

When the cooking is done, manually release the pressure and remove the lid. Transfer the meat to a large bowl and shred or cut into pieces.

Add the xanthan gum to the broth inside the Crock-Pot Express and return the meat. Stir the parsley and allow to heat through. Serve and enjoy!

Nutrition:

Calories: 393

Fat: 28g

Carbohydrates: 4g

Dietary Fiber: 1g

Protein: 30g

Oozing Ground Beef Shawarma

Preparation Time: 5 minutes

Cooking Time: 20 minutes

Servings: 4

Ingredients:

1 pound of lean ground beef

1 cup of onions, sliced

1 cup of red peppers, thickly sliced

2 cups of cabbage, chopped

2 tablespoons of shawarma mix

1 teaspoon of salt

Directions:

Press the "Sautee/Browning" button on the Crock-Pot Express and add the ground beef. Cook until the beef is brown, breaking up the meat into smaller bits using a metal or wooden spoon.

Add the onions, red peppers, cabbage, shawarma mix, and salt to the Crock-Pot Express. Stir until well combined.

Lock the lid and ensure the valve is closed.

Press the "Meat/Stew" button and set the time to 2 minutes.

When the cooking is done, naturally release the pressure for 5 minutes, then manually release the remaining pressure. Remove the lid.

Serve and enjoy!

Nutrition:

Calories: 191

Fat: 5g

Carbohydrates: 8g

Dietary Fiber: 2g

Protein: 25g

Full-Flavored Pot Roast

Preparation Time: 10 minutes

Cooking Time: 45 minutes

Servings: 8

Ingredients:

2 tablespoons of avocado oil

1 (4 pounds) beef pot roast, cut into large chunks

1 cup of beef broth

1 teaspoon of smoked paprika

1 teaspoon of onion powder

1 teaspoon of garlic powder

1 teaspoon of salt

1 teaspoon of black pepper

1 teaspoon of xanthan gum

Directions:

Press the "Sautee/Browning" button on the Crock-Pot Express and add the avocado oil.

Once hot, add the roast and brown on both sides. Remove and set aside.

Deglaze the Crock-Pot Express with the beef broth and scrape any browned bits from the bottom of the pot.

Return the roast to the Crock-Pot Express and season with salt, paprika, onion powder, garlic powder, salt, and black pepper.

Lock the lid and ensure the valve is closed.

Press the "Meat/Stew" button and set the time to 35 minutes. Press start.

When the cooking is done, naturally release the pressure and remove the lid.

Transfer the roast to a plate.

Sprinkle the xanthan gum to the liquid and stir until thickens. Return the roast to the liquid and stir until coated. Serve and enjoy!

Nutrition:

Calories: 427

Fat: 14.6g

Carbohydrates: 0.2g

Dietary Fiber: 0.2g

Protein: 68.2g

Generous Mongolian Beef

Preparation Time: 5 minutes

Cooking Time: 17 minutes

Servings: 4

Ingredients:

1 pound of beef, thinly sliced

¼ teaspoon of salt

½ teaspoon of black pepper

1 tablespoon of olive oil

¼ cup of light brown sugar

¼ cup of soy sauce

2 garlic cloves, minced

2 tablespoons of sweet chili sauce

¼ teaspoon of ground ginger

1 tablespoon of xanthan gum

Directions:

In a bowl, add the soy sauce, brown sugar, garlic, sweet chili sauce, ginger, and xanthan gum. Mix well and set aside.

Press the "Saute/Browning" button on the Crock-Pot Express and add the olive oil.

Once hot, working in batches, add the beef and cook for 1 minute per side. Remove and set aside.

Return all the cooked beef slices to the Crock-Pot Express and add the sauce.

Cook until the sauce thickens with the beef.

Serve and enjoy!

Nutrition:

Calories: 317

Fat: 11.2g

Carbohydrates: 15.9g

Dietary Fiber: 1.7g

Protein: 36.3g

French Onion Meatloaf

Preparation Time: 10 minutes

Cooking Time: 1 hour and 30 minutes

Servings: 8

Ingredients:

Caramelized Ingredients:

2 onions, thinly sliced

4 tablespoons of unsalted butter

French Onion Meatloaf Ingredients:

2 pounds of ground beef

1 tablespoon of olive oil

½ cup of crushed saltines

½ cup of caramelized onions

1 large egg

2 teaspoons of salt

1 tablespoon of fresh thyme

1 teaspoon of black pepper

½ teaspoon of red pepper flakes

½ cup of beef stock

Gruyere Gravy Ingredients:

2 tablespoons of almond or coconut flour

¾ cup of beef stock

1 tablespoon of fresh thyme

½ cup of gruyere cheese, shredded

Directions:

Press the "Sautee/Browning" button on the Crock-Pot Express and add the butter.

Once the butter is melted, add the onions and cook until brown and caramelized, stirring constantly.

Turn off "Sautee/Browning" button on the Crock-Pot Express and transfer to a plate. Allow to cool and set aside.

In a large bowl, add all the meatloaf ingredients EXCEPT for the olive oil and beef stock and stir until well combined. Form into one or two loaves.

Press the "Sautee/Browning" button on the Crock-Pot Express and add the olive oil.

Once hot, add the loaves and sauté until brown.

Once hot, add the loaf(s) and brown on all sides. Add the beef stock to the Crock-Pot Express. Lock the lid and ensure the valve is closed.

Press the "Meat/Stew" button on the Crock-Pot Express and set the time to 18 minutes. Press start.

When the cooking is done, naturally release the pressure and remove the lid. Remove the meatloaf.

Press "Sautee/Browning" button on the Crock-Pot Express and add the almond or coconut flour to the Crock-Pot Express.

Add the reserved caramelized onions, fresh thyme, cheese, and beef stock to the Crock-Pot Express.

Ladle the sauce over the meatloaf. Serve and enjoy!

Nutrition:

Calories: 421

Fat: 32g

Carbohydrates: 9g

Dietary Fiber: 1g

Protein: 24g

Classy Corned Beef

Preparation Time: 10 minutes

Cooking Time: 1 hour and 45 minutes

Servings: 8

Ingredients:

3 pounds of corned beef brisket

2 bay leaves

3 garlic cloves, peeled

1 onion, quartered

Water, as needed

Directions:

Add the beef brisket, bay leaves, garlic cloves, and onions to the Crock-Pot Express.

Pour enough water to cover the brisket.

Lock the lid and ensure the valve is closed.

Press the "Meat/Stew" button and cook at High Pressure for 90 minutes.

When the cooking is done, naturally release the pressure for 10 minutes, then manually release the remaining pressure. Remove the lid.

Transfer the corned beef to a serving platter and shred using two forks.

Serve and enjoy!

Nutrition:

Calories: 238

Fat: 8.1g

Carbohydrates: 0g

Dietary Fiber: 0g

Protein: 38.7g

Signature Salsa Pork Chops

Preparation Time: 5 minutes

Cooking Time: 20 minutes

Servings: 6

Ingredients:

6 bone-in pork chops

1 teaspoon of salt

1 teaspoon of black pepper

3 tablespoons of olive oil

1 (24-ounce) jar of chunky salsa

Directions:

Season the pork chops with salt and black pepper.

Press the "Sautee/Browning" button on the Crock-Pot Express and add the olive oil.

Once hot, working in batches, add the pork chops and cook until brown on each side. Remove and set aside.

Add all the pork chops to the cooking pot and pour the jar of chunky salsa over.

Lock the lid and ensure the valve is closed.

Press the "Meat/Stew" button on the Crock-Pot Express and set the time to 8 minutes.

When the cooking is done, naturally release the pressure and remove the lid.

Transfer the pork chops to serving plates and top with salsa from the Crock-Pot Express.

Serve and enjoy!

Nutrition:

Calories: 347

Fat: 27.1g

Carbohydrates: 7.1g

Dietary Fiber: 1.8g

Protein: 19.7g

Chicken Adobo

Preparation Time: 10 minutes

Cooking Time: 40 minutes

Servings: 4

Ingredients:

4 chicken legs, thighs, and drumsticks separated

2 tablespoons of coconut oil

1/3 cup of soy sauce

¼ cup of granulated erythritol

¼ cup of distilled white vinegar

5 garlic cloves, crushed

2 dried bay leaves

1 large yellow onion, sliced

2 scallions, sliced

1 teaspoon of salt

1 teaspoon of black pepper

Directions:

Season the chicken legs with salt and black pepper.

Press "Sautee/Browning" on your Crock-Pot Express and add the coconut oil.

Once the oil is hot, add the chicken and brown on both sides, about 7 minutes. You may need to work in batches.

Return all the chicken to the Crock-Pot Express and stir in the soy sauce, granulated Erythritol, distilled white vinegar, 5 crushed garlic cloves, 2 dried bay leaves, 1 sliced large yellow onion, salt, and black pepper.

Lock the lid and ensure the valve is closed.

Press the "Poultry" button and set the time to 8 minutes. Press start.

When the cooking is done, manually release the pressure and remove the lid.

Press "Sautee/Browning" button and bring to a boil. Boil and reduce the liquid until dark brown and fragrant, about 20 minutes, stirring occasionally. Remove the bay leaves.

Transfer the chicken to a serving plate and ladle the sauce over.

Sprinkle with scallions. Serve and enjoy!

Nutrition:

Calories: 356

Fat: 17.7g

Carbohydrates: 8g

Dietary Fiber: 0.3g

Protein: 43.8g

Parmesan Garlic Nut Chicken Wings

Preparation Time: 15 minutes

Cooking Time: 4 hours

Ingredients:

½ cup / 100 g of chicken wings

1/2 tablespoon / 7 gr chopped garlic

1 tablespoons / 14 gr olive oil

2 tablespoons / 28 gr of ghee

1 tablespoon / 14 gr of mayonnaise

1 tablespoon / 14 gr of Stevia

1 tablespoon / 14 gr grated Parmesan cheese, grated

1 teaspoon / 5 gr of lemon juice

1 teaspoon / 5 gr of apple cider vinegar

1 pinch of dry oregano

1 pinch of dried basil

Salt, pepper and chili pepper to taste

Fresh basil or parsley (to embellish)

1 pinch xanthan gum optional thickener

Directions:

The first thing to do is prepare the sauce. All the ingredients, except for the chicken, must be mixed together in a large bowl.

Then smear the Slow Cooker with a little butter or a non-sticking spray.

Then pour half the sauce on the bottom. Add the chicken wings and cover

Cook in the Slow Cooker with the lid at HIGH temperature for 4 hours

Gently take out one by one the chicken wings from the Slow Cooker and place them on a baking tray covered with aluminum foil.

Pour the left over sauce on the wings (spread the sauce over the chicken by using a kitchen brush or a spoon) and bake in the oven on grill mode for another 15 minutes at about 200 degrees C / 390 degrees F to get a crunchy crust

Serve the chicken wings topped with garlic and parmesan while it's still hot

Nutrition:

Calories: 575.88 Kcal

Fat: 48.14 g

Total carbs: 0.1

Net carbs: 0.1

Protein 37.04 g

Tikka Masala Chicken

Preparation Time: 15 minutes

Cooking Time: 4 hours

Ingredients:

½ cup / 100 gr of chicken breast

2 tablespoons / 28 gr of tomato sauce

2 tablespoons / 28 gr of coconut milk

1 teaspoon / 5 gr of fresh ginger

1 pinch of onion powder

1 clove / 3 gr of garlic

1 teaspoon / 5 gr of thickener (Xanatum gum)

2 tablespoons / 28 gr of olive oil

1 tablespoon / 28 gr of cocoa butter

1 tablespoon of garam masala

1 pinch of cumin powder

1 pinch of salt

1 pinch of curcuma

1 pinch of ground black pepper

1 pinch of paprika

1 pinch of fresh coriander

1 dash of lemon juice

Directions:

Rinse the chicken breast leaving the skin and cut it into cubes of about 3 cm

With your hands, grease the chicken cubes all around in the cocoa butter so to soften the meat uniformly

Clean and chop the garlic and ginger. Regarding the ginger, you can also leave it in bigger pieces and remove it at the end of the cooking if you do not wish to eat it, otherwise chop it finely

Combine all spices and salt

At this point, combine all the ingredients into the Slow Cooker, with the chicken and cover with tomato sauce, coconut milk, olive oil and lemon juice

Stir well for the whole so as to season the meat evenly.

Turn the Slow Cooker on HIGH and cook for 4 hours

Half an hour before the end of the cooking add a tablespoon of thickener, to thicken the cooking broth, and stir well to avoid lumps

Garnish it all with crushed fresh coriander

Nutrition:

Calories: 596 Kcal

Fat: 49 g

Total carbs: 5

Net carbs: 5

Protein 33 g

Hot Spicy Chicken

Preparation Time: 15 minutes

Cooking Time: 3 hours

Ingredients:

½ cup / 100 gr of chicken

2 tablespoons / 28 gr of olive oil

1 tablespoon / 14 gr of fresh ginger root

1 tablespoon / 14 gr of white onion, sliced

1 tablespoon / 14 gr of coco butter

1 teaspoon / 5 gr of rosemary needles

1 pinch of salt

Directions:

Remove the skin from the chicken

Cut the onion in slices, and roll it with your hands into the cocoa butter to soften

Clean and divide the ginger in 2 parts (this will make it easier to locate it and remove it at the end of cooking)

Put all the ingredients in the pot, adding salt and rosemary

Cover it with oil, and mix the ingredients well

Although the chicken will not be completely covered it is not a problem, it will cook correctly

Turn the pot on HIGH for 3 hours

After half of the cooking time, turn the chicken over, especially if it is not completely covered with oil

After cooking, pour over the chicken a bit of the stew liquid. The chicken will be uniquely soft

Nutrition:

Calories: 502

Fat: 45 g

Total carbs: 4

Net carbs: 4

Protein 32 g

Savory Duck Breast

Preparation Time: 15 minutes

Cooking Time: 5 hours

Ingredients:

½ cup / 100 gr of duck breast

2 tablespoons / 28 gr of pine nuts

1 tablespoon / 14 gr of fresh plums, diced

2 tablespoons / 28 gr of carrot, diced

1 pinch of onion powder

2 tablespoons / 28 gr of celery stalk, diced

2 tablespoons / 28 gr of ghee

1 pinch of fresh basil, chopped

1 pinch of chili powder

1 pinch of salt

For the dip:

2 tablespoons / 28 gr of mayonnaise

1 pinch of chili powder

Directions:

Open the duck breast by placing the inside upward, season with salt and pepper and a dash of oil

Chop all the vegetables together and mix together with the pine nuts, ghee and plums, and put them on the bottom of the Slow Cooker

If you have a grid, put it in the pot over the vegetables and lay on it the duck

Set the Slow Cooker on HIGH and cook for 5 hours

When finished cooking, remove the chest from the pot and place it on a plate, remove the skin that should be easily removable at this point

At this point you can use the seasoning and pour it over the meat. Garnish with some basil leaves

Nutrition:

Calories: 742

Fat: 54

Total carbs: 7.5

Net carbs: 7.5

Protein 27.2 g

Autumn Sweet Chicken

Preparation Time: 15 minutes

Cooking Time: 5 hours

Ingredients:

3 tablespoons / 36 gr of Stevia powder

2 tablespoons / 28 gr of walnuts, roasted

1 pinch of ground cinnamon

1 pinch of ground nutmeg

1 pinch of ground turmeric

A pinch of salt

1 boneless and skinless chicken leg

2 tablespoons / 28 gr olive oil

2 tablespoons / 28 gr ghee

1 pinch of onion powder

1 dash of lemon juice

33 cc / 1 fl oz of chicken broth

1 pinch of rosemary

½ cinnamon stick

Directions:

Roast the walnuts in a frying pan. Remove from the stove and set aside to cool

Divide in half and use a blender to crumble half of them

Mix the Stevia, ground cinnamon, turmeric, nutmeg, and salt in a large bowl. Add the skinless chicken and roll it so it is covered evenly

Heat a frying pan and sauté the chicken until golden

Dissolve the butter in the same pan on medium heat. Add the onions powder, chopped nuts, lemon juice, and broth, into your Slow Cooker pot with a spoon. Add the spicy chicken and the remaining spice mixture

Add by mixing the garlic clove, rosemary and cinnamon stick

Cover and cook on LOW for 5 hours

Nutrition:

Calories: 687

Fat: 63 gr

Total carbs: 5

Net carbs: 3

Protein 25 g

Coconut & Basil Chicken

Preparation Time: 15 minutes

Cooking Time: 4 hours

Ingredients:

½ cup / 100 gr of skinless and boneless chicken

33 cc / 1 fl oz of coconut milk

2 tablespoons / 28 gr of ghee

1 tablespoon / 14 gr of fresh basil leaves

1 teaspoon / 5 gr of chopped ginger

1 clove / 3 gr of garlic

1 dash of lime juice

1 pinch of cumin

For the dip:

2 tablespoons of olive oil

1 tablespoon / 14 gr of grated coconut, dehydrated

1 pinch of curry

1 pinch of salt

1 pinch of fresh basil, chopped

Directions:

Prepare the chicken sauce combining the coconut milk, basil, ginger, garlic, lime juice, cumin, curry, salt, pepper and cinnamon in a mixer. Mix until it's well combined

In the meantime prepare the dip: combine all dip ingredients mixing well. Put aside to chill for a few hours so the flavors enriches

Lay the skinless and boneless chicken in the Slow Cooker. Pour the sauce over the chicken and cook for 4 hours on HIGH

When the chicken is tender and well-cooked separate it from the sauce

Pour the sauce into a saucepan and heat it on the stove for a few minutes to make it denser, before pouring over the chicken on a plate

Nutrition:

Calories: 605.9

Fat: 55.2 g

Total carbs: 5.61

Net carbs: 3.37

Protein 22.4 g

Cheesy Chicken Pot

Preparation Time: 15 minutes

Cooking Time: 8 hours

Ingredients:

¼ cup / 100 gr of skinless and boneless chicken

2 tablespoons / 28 gr of white onion, chopped

2 tablespoons / 28 gr of carrots, finely chopped

1 tablespoon / 14 gr of Cheddar cheese, diced

2 tablespoons / 28 gr of ghee

1 pinch of oregano

1 pinch of time

1 tablespoon / 14 gr of cocoa butter

¼ cup / 100 gr of sour cream

Directions:

Pour all of your ingredients in the Slow Cooker pot, except for the sour cream, cocoa butter, and Cheddar and ghee

Cover and cook on LOW for 8 hours and pour the sour cream, cheddar and ghee in

Cook for another half an hour without the lid

Nutrition:

Calories: 590

Fat: 50 g

Total carbs: 5.5

Net carbs: 5.5

Protein 35 g

Beijing Chicken Soup

Preparation Time: 20 minutes

Cooking Time: 4 hours

Ingredients:

¼ cup / 100 gr of finely chopped chicken scallops

33 cc / 1 fl oz chicken broth

2 tablespoons / 28 gr of shitake mushrooms, minced

1 tablespoon / 14 gr of fresh grated ginger

2 tablespoons / 28 gr of carrots, julienne cut

2 tablespoons / 28 gr of ghee

2 tablespoons / 28 gr of olive oil

1 pinch of garlic powder

1 heart of lemongrass stem, crushed

1 tablespoon / 14 gr of spicy soy sauce

1 pinch of fresh chopped coriander

33 cc / 1 fl oz of water

1 pinch of salt

Directions:

Pour in your Slow Cooker pot the vegetables, chicken minced mushrooms, ginger and garlic

Add the water, broth, lemongrass, soy sauce and coriander

Cover and cook on LOW for 4 hours

Nutrition:

Calories: 610

Fat: 55 gr

Total carbs: 7.5

Net carbs: 7.5

Protein 36 g